Donald k. Cilley

FOREVER CHEMICAL AND PERFLUOOCTANE SULFATE

How damage chemical cause to the liver

First edition

This book was professionally typeset on Reedsy
Find out more at reedsy.com

Contents

INTRODUCTION

Humans typically live for 80 years. However, the lifespan of the cells that comprise our body is substantially shorter (for example, skin – 2 weeks, liver – 400 days). New cells emerge after the death of the old ones.

Cancer

a term for illnesses in which unusual cells can assault nearby tissues by segregating uncontrollably. Additionally, disease cells can move to various body regions via the blood and lymphatic systems. Malignant growth comes in a few main forms. A condition called carcinoma begins in the skin or in the tissues that surround or border internal organs. Beginning in bone, ligament, fat, muscle, veins, or other connective or stable tissue, sarcoma is a disease. Leukemia is a condition that develops in bone marrow or other blood-forming tissue and causes an abnormally high production of platelets. Tumors like lymphoma and other myelomas begin in the cells of the immune system. Focal sensory system malignant growths are conditions that begin in the brain and spinal cord tissues. also known as peril.

What causes cancer?

In essence, cancer cells are cells that have undergone a number of mutations and reached a stage where they can grow/replicate quickly and uncontrollably. They have become immortal, these cells.

Because these mutations don't build up in a single original cell at once, but rather in a cell lineage over time, cancer is frequently a slow-moving, sneaky disease.

One cell may experience a single mutation, and all of that cell's progeny will carry that mutation. Then one of those cells acquires a second mutation, resulting in two mutations in all of that cell's progeny. And so on, and so forth, until you have cell children with enough mutations to get around your body's many regulatory mechanisms and proliferate quickly. This is how cancer cells clonally evolve.

These mutations are merely DNA faults that can be brought on by either internal (such as hormones, genetics from your parents, metabolic or autoimmune diseases) or external (such as environmental) influences (e.g. chemicals, radiation, smoking, infections, etc).

There are six basic characteristics that are frequently linked to malignant cells;

Insensitive to anti-growth signals, they are capable of producing their own growth signals.

They avoid the "apoptosis" that normal cells experience when their DNA is broken or programmed cell death.

They can stimulate the growth of new blood artery branches to feed them with nutrients. They have replicative immortality (normal cells have a limited number of replications until they can no longer divide; cancer cells can overcome this by producing specific enzymes).

Malignant cancer cells can invade and spread to other tissues through a process called metastasis.

Cancerous cells develop these skills over time as a result of a steady accumulation of DNA errors or mutations.

There are typically two primary categories of mutation.

A gain-of-function mutation will add new functionality to the cell. For instance, the growth factor receptors on cells await a signal from the surrounding environment. When they become active, they instruct the cell to start the cell cycle and divide. Cancerous cells can occasionally have a mutation in this receptor that makes it permanently turned on, allowing them to cycle through the cell cycle repeatedly and divide quickly.

Normal genes that aid in a cell's growth and development are referred to as proto-oncogenes, and when they acquire gain-of-function mutations, they are referred to as oncogenes. We have two copies of each gene, and a proto-oncogene can become an oncogene by undergoing a gain-of-function mutation in just one copy.

Also known as tumour suppressor genes, these genes are designed to stop cells from growing out of control. They do this by identifying DNA damage, halting the cell cycle to repair the damage, or, in the case of damage that cannot be repaired, by inducing cell suicide. These tumor suppressor genes are inactivated by mutations that occur in cancer cells, or "knock out" the genes. These changes are referred to as loss-of-function mutations, and when a tumour suppressor gene is inactive, it is unable to prevent an uncontrollably expanding cell.

Since a single mutation only affects one copy of the gene, the other copy will still function and be able to repair DNA damage, you need two loss-of-function mutations (one in each copy of the tumour suppressor gene) to eradicate it.

PFOS

Researchers from the USC Keck School of Medicine have found that the common polyfluoroalkyl substance (PFAS) may increase the risk of liver cancer.

Recent studies have linked non-viral hepatocellular carcinoma, the most frequent kind of liver cancer, to exposure to a synthetic chemical that is commonly present in the environment.

The compound, also known as perfluooctane sulfate (PFOS), belongs to a group of synthetic chemicals termed per- and polyfluoroalkyl substances (PFAS). Because they degrade very slowly and build up in the environment and human tissue, including the liver, these chemicals are used in a wide range of consumer and commercial products. This is why they are frequently referred to as "forever chemicals."

According to earlier animal studies, exposure to PFAS increases the incidence of liver cancer. However, this is the initial investigation to use human samples to support a relationship.

Jesse Goodrich, PhD, a postdoctoral scholar in the Department of Population and Public Health Sciences at the Keck School of Medicine, said, "This builds on the prior study but takes it one step further." This is the first study in people to demonstrate a link between PFAS and liver cancer, which is one of the most devastating outcomes of liver illness.

More exposure means more risk.

The research team from the Keck School of Medicine used human samples that were gathered as part of a sizable epidemiological investigation. More than 200,000 inhabitants of Los Angeles and Hawaii have been monitored as part of the Multiethnic Cohort Study, a project that was developed in partnership between the medical school and the University of Hawaii.

The research team was able to identify 50 volunteers who later acquired liver cancer and assess the blood samples collected before their cancer diagnosis thanks to this extensive collection of human blood and tissue samples. Additionally, they were able to contrast them with 50 individuals from the same researchers who did not get cancer.

You need the correct samples, which is part of the reason there haven't been many human studies, according to Veronica Wendy Setiawan, PhD, a professor of population and public health sciences at the Keck School of Medicine. Because cancer takes time to develop, samples must be collected far before a diagnosis when examining an environmental exposure.

The blood samples that were drawn prior to the person developing liver cancer included numerous different kinds of PFAS, according to researchers. According to the study, there is a substantial link between PFOS and liver cancer. Additionally, research revealed that those with the highest blood levels of PFOS had a 4.5-fold higher risk of developing liver cancer than those with the lowest levels.

A Chemical interferes with proper liver function

The research team was also able to provide light on potential ways that PFOS affected the liver's typical function. As a result of their analysis of the samples, they discovered proof that PFOS may affect the liver's regular processes for metabolizing glucose, bile acids, and branched-chain amino acids.

More fat may build up in the liver as a result of disturbed regular metabolic functions. NAFLD, also known as non-alcoholic fatty liver disease, is the name of this ailment. Globally, NAFLD has recently increased dramatically and for no apparent reason. This is particularly troubling because liver cancer is far more likely to occur in those with NAFLD.

By 2030, it is anticipated that 30% of American adults would have NAFLD.

increasing awareness of PFAS exposure's consequences on health

PFAS, which are present in many consumer and industrial items, were first found in the blood of workers who had been exposed to them at work in the 1970s. They were discovered in the blood of the general public in the 1990s, which raised awareness of the potential health dangers.

The use of PFOA and PFOS has been phased out by several manufacturers. However, because they persist for a long time, PFAS are found in more than 98% of adult Americans' blood, many food products, and drinking water.

The majority of the studies on the associations between PFAS exposure and liver damage, liver illness, and now liver cancer have been carried out by researchers at the Keck School of Medicine, under the direction of Leda Chatzi, MD, PhD, professor of population and public health sciences. In a larger study planned for later this year, they intend to further validate their findings regarding the connection with liver cancer.

According to Chatzi, "We think our work offers significant new understandings into the long-term health implications that these chemicals have on human health, particularly with respect to how they can impair normal liver function." This work closes a critical gap in our knowledge of the actual effects of chemical exposure.

Children's Hepatoblastoma (Liver Cancer): Signs and Treatment

How Does Liver Cancer Occur?

Though approximately 2 to 3 persons in a million are affected, hepatoblastoma is the most frequent liver cancer in children. Children are affected within the first three years of life, and it typically manifests as an abdominal tumor that hurts and is uncomfortable. These tumors commonly affect young children who were born prematurely. With surgical removal, the tumor can be cured. The tumor's size and location within the liver make surgical removal risky, but liver transplantation can still treat the condition.

How pediatric liver cancer treated

According to estimates, a liver transplant may be necessary for one in five hepatoblastoma tumors. Additionally, hepatoblastoma now represents 7.5% of all pediatric liver transplants, compared to less than 3% for other pediatric liver malignancies. Chemotherapy is started as soon as a diagnosis is made and is continued following a liver transplant. If the tumor is limited to the liver, up to 80% of children who receive liver transplants survive more than 20 years without recurrence.

After transplantation, 16% of children may experience recurrences. Recurrences are more frequent in the first two years and uncommon beyond that. Lungs are where hepatoblastoma most frequently metastasizes. It's interesting to note that even when the tumor is outside the liver, removing it by surgery or chemotherapy prior to transplantation can still cure up to 50% of these kids.

Children with hepatoblastoma must be referred for surgery and/or transplantation as soon as possible due to the possibility of a cure, even if the tumor has spread outside the liver or if it is particularly large.

Who is predisposed to liver cancer

It is imperative to definitively separate hepatoblastoma from the more prevalent hepatocellular carcinoma. Adults can develop hepatocellular carcinoma, which typically strikes those who already have cirrhosis or infectious hepatitis and do not react well to chemotherapy. Large tumors that enter blood arteries or have expanded outside the liver have a terrible prognosis for survival. One might easily infer that a large hepatoblastoma that invades blood vessels or has moved to a single place beyond the liver is inoperable since it presumably acts like the "normal" liver cancer because there is so much more information regarding hepatocellular carcinoma.

Numerous investigations from various institutions have demonstrated that this is untrue. Hepatoblastoma of a more basic variety known as "anaplastic" is treated differently from other types of hepatoblastoma through liver transplantation. The majority of times after this sort of hepatoblastoma has been surgically removed, it returns to the liver. Recurrences of this form of hepatoblastoma were neither more nor less common among the 35 children with the disease who had treatment at the Hillman Center for Pediatric Transplantation at Children's Hospital of Pittsburgh of UPMC.

Working with a knowledgeable hematologist-oncologist who specializes in treating children with liver cancer is thus the best course of action if hepatoblastoma has been identified. The Pediatric Cooperative Oncology Group has tested great chemotherapy regimens during the past ten years. Pediatric oncologists can carry out these procedures while making referrals for tumor removal by surgery or transplantation.

Children's Liver Cancer Symptoms

Children's liver cancer symptoms are frequently hazy and go unrecognized. Symptoms of liver cancer include the following:

-reduced appetite
  -Unaccounted-for weight loss
  -Fever
  -Fatigues \Weakness
  -abdominal pain
  -enlarged abdomen
  -Nausea
  -dark feces-
  -Skin or eye whites that have become yellow

Other, less serious medical disorders may also be at blame for these symptoms. Anyone displaying these signs ought to visit a physician.

diagnosis of childhood liver cancer

A physical examination is the first step in the diagnosis of hepatoblastoma, after which the doctor will go over your child's symptoms and medical history. The doctor will advise testing to confirm or rule out the diagnosis if they have a suspicion of liver cancer. Testing might involve:

Blood tests - These can check the health of your child's liver or look for markers in the blood that suggest the presence of liver cancer. Alpha-fetoprotein (AFP), a substance produced by the majority of hepatoblastomas and some hepatocellular carcinomas, is released into the bloodstream. Doctors can sometimes determine if a child's cancer is responding to treatment by checking the levels of AFP in the child's blood.

X-rays of the abdomen and chest

Blood vessel X-rays are known as angiograms.

A procedure called an MRI scan uses magnetic waves to create images of the liver's inside.

Ultrasound is another test that employs high-frequency sound waves to produce images of the liver and other interior organs.

Using a computer and X-ray technology, a CT scan creates images of the liver inside.

Laparoscopy: A small incision in the belly is made, and a thin, lit tube is inserted to view the liver.

In a biopsy, a sample of liver tissue is removed to look for cancerous cells. usually carried out through a laparoscopic operation or utilizing a specific hollow needle.

Stages of liver cancer

Additional tests will be performed after liver cancer has been identified to determine whether cancer cells have spread to other bodily regions. Because they need to determine what stage the cancer is in, doctors refer to this process as "staging." The doctors for your child can then arrange the most effective course of treatment once they have this information. The phases utilized for pediatric liver cancer are as follows:

Liver cancer at stage I is curable by surgery.

Stage II Liver Cancer – The majority of cancer may be eliminated after surgery, but a very tiny quantity of cancer (microscopically small levels) may remain in the liver.

Stage III liver cancer – Some of the cancer may be surgically removed, but some of the tumors may stay in the lymph nodes or the abdomen.

Stage IV liver cancer: cancer has metastasized outside of the liver.

Liver cancer that has returned (or recurred) after treatment is referred to as recurrent liver cancer. It could recur in the liver or somewhere else in the body.

Treatment for pediatric liver cancer

Treatments for pediatric liver cancer are determined by the kind (hepatoblastoma or hepatocellular carcinoma) and stage of the disease, as well as the age and overall condition of the kid.

Surgery may be done to remove the malignancy and the affected portion of the liver. Cancer that has spread to other body parts may potentially be removed through surgery.

Liver transplantation may be a possibility for some individuals with earlier stages of liver cancer, particularly hepatocellular carcinoma. The liver can be replaced by surgery with a healthy liver from a donor. If this option is a viable treatment, the doctor for your kid will talk about it with you.

Drugs are used in chemotherapy to kill cancer cells. Chemotherapy may be administered to your child either prior to surgery to help shrink the liver cancer or afterward to eradicate any leftover cells. Adjuvant chemotherapy is the type of chemotherapy used after surgery when cancer has been removed by the doctor. Chemotherapy for pediatric liver cancer is often administered by inserting a needle into an artery or vein. Because the medicine enters the bloodstream, circulates throughout the body, and has the ability to eradicate cancer cells outside of the liver, this type of chemotherapy is referred to as systemic therapy. Drugs are injected directly into the blood arteries that supply the liver during direct infusion chemotherapy, another type of chemotherapy.

For the treatment of pediatric liver cancer, a unique procedure known as chemo-embolization is occasionally employed. In order to prevent or slow the blood flow into the malignancy, chemotherapy medications are injected into the liver's major artery. As a result, the medications take longer to destroy the cancer cells, and the cancer cells are also kept from obtaining the oxygen and nutrition they require to thrive.

X-rays and other powerful rays are used in radiation therapy to destroy cancer cells and reduce tumor size. Radiation may be administered by small plastic tubes placed in the region with the cancer cells or through a machine placed outside the body (external radiation therapy) (internal radiation therapy).

Biological therapy, also known as biological response modifier (BRM) therapy, is a form of cancer treatment that makes use of drugs or naturally occurring chemicals to boost or restore the body's natural defenses against the disease.

After the course of treatment is complete, your kid will get routine scans, chest X-rays, and blood tests to check the amount of alpha-fetoprotein (if necessary). This enables the medical professionals caring for your kid to track the efficacy of the therapy and identify any early cancer recurrences.

Your child's prognosis, which includes the likelihood of recovery, is based on the stage of the liver cancer, specifically whether or not it has spread, the histology, or how the cancer cells appear under a microscope, as well as your child's general health. Like with most cancers, children have considerably higher cure rates than adults do. More than half of children with hepatoblastoma are cured, and the prognosis is much better for those who only have tiny tumors in the liver.

Symptoms of prostate chemicals

Although it is a frequent kind of cancer in men, prostate cancer is very treatable in its early stages. The prostate gland, which is located between the penis and the bladder, is where it starts.

The prostate serves a number of purposes. These include releasing PSA, a protein that helps semen maintain its liquid state, generating the fluid that nourishes and transports sperm, and assisting with urinary control.

Prostate cancer is the most prevalent cancer affecting men in the United States, aside from skin cancer. According to the American Cancer Society (ACS), there will be roughly 34,130 prostate cancer fatalities and 248,530 new cases of prostate cancer in 2021.

Prostate cancer will be diagnosed in about 1 in 8 men at some time in their lives. But only 1 in 41 of them will pass away as a result. This is due to the fact that treatment, especially early treatment, is beneficial. The majority of prostate cancer cases can be found by doctors through routine screening before they spread.

Symptoms and signs

Early prostate cancer frequently has no symptoms, but screening might find alterations that can be cancerous. Using a test, screeningTrusted Source can determine how much PSA is present in the blood. High levels imply the possibility of malignancy.

Men who do have symptoms might notice

dependable source

inability to begin and maintain urinating
a persistent urge to urinate, particularly at night, a weak urine stream, and blood or semen in the urine
back, hips, or pelvic pain during urination or ejaculation
advanced signs
Advanced prostate cancer patients may also go undiagnosed. cancer's size and the extent of its internal dissemination will determine any potential symptoms. The following signs and symptoms of advanced prostate cancer can also be present:

fatigue, undiagnosed weight loss, and bone discomfort

Treatment

Treatment will depend on the stage of cancer, as well as other elements including the Gleason score and PSA levels. Several treatment approaches may be appropriate regardless of the stage of cancer, it is also important to note.

We list a few possible treatments in the sections that follow.

Explore what treatment options for prostate cancer can entail for fertility at a reliable source.

prostate cancer in its early stages
Depending on how little and limited the cancer is, a doctor might advise:

monitoring or waiting with vigilance
Regular PSA blood levels may be checked by the doctor, but no immediate action will be taken. The risk of therapy adverse effects may exceed the necessity for rapid treatment because prostate cancer develops slowly.

Surgery
To remove the tumor, a surgeon may perform a radical prostatectomy. The surgery may include the removal of the prostate as well as the surrounding tissue, seminal vesicles,

and neighboring lymph nodes. This operation can be carried out by a medical professional either by open, laparoscopic, or robot-assisted laparoscopic surgery.

radiation treatment

Radiation is used in this to either kill or stop the growth of cancer cells. Options for prostate cancer in its early stages include dependable source

External radiation therapy: This treatment sends radiation to the cancer cells from a machine outside the body. A type of external radiation known as conformal radiation therapy employs a computer to help guide and target a particular spot, reducing the risk to healthy tissue and enabling a high dose of radiation to reach the prostate tumor.

Internal radiation therapy, also known as brachytherapy, is a treatment that involves the implantation of radioactive seeds close to the prostate by a physician. A surgeon utilizes imaging tests like computed tomography or ultrasound to assist in directing where to place the radioactive material.

Treatment will depend on a number of variables. A doctor will talk about the person's best course of action.

prostate cancer that has spread.

Cancer can spread throughout the body as it becomes worse. Treatment choices may alter if it spreads or if it returns after remission. Options consist of:

Chemotherapy: This treatment approach makes use of medications to slow the spread of cancer cells. Although it can eradicate cancer cells all over the body, there could be negative effects from it.

Androgens are male hormones used in hormonal therapy. Testosterone and dihydrotestosterone are the two primary androgens. The proliferation of cancer cells appears to be stopped or delayed by blocking or decreasing these hormones. One choice is to have the testicles, which are responsible for producing most of the body's hormones, surgically removed. Other medications may be helpful.

Immunotherapy: This treatment makes use of the immune system to combat cancer. To assist strengthen or restore the body's natural defenses against cancer, scientists can employ compounds the body makes or make them in a lab.

Targeted therapy: This technique employs medications or other chemicals that recognize and kill particular cancer cells. For instance, a study from 2021 spotlights a radiopharmaceutical treatment strategy that could be successful for difficult-to-treat kinds of advanced prostate cancer.

effects on conceiving

There is a role for the prostate gland in sexual reproduction. Fertility is impacted in a variety of ways by prostate cancer and many of its therapies.

For instance, fertility and semen output will be impacted by surgery to remove either the prostate gland or the testicles. Additionally, radiation therapy can harm prostate tissue, sperm, and the volume of semen needed to deliver it. Treatment with hormones may potentially impact fertility.

But there are ways to keep these processes intact, such as sperm banking before surgery or sperm extraction from the testicles themselves for artificial insemination.

After prostate cancer therapy, fertility is not guaranteed to be unaffected. When developing a treatment plan, patients who wish to become parents following treatment should talk with their doctor about their fertility choices.

Causes

The precise cause of prostate cancer is unknown to researchers. It develops when particular alterations take place, typically in glandular cells. Prostatic intraepithelial neoplasia is the term a doctor may use to describe alterations in prostate gland cells (PIN). Nearly half of all men over 50 have a PIN, according to a reliable source.

The cells won't be malignant at first, and the changes will be gradual. They might eventually develop cancer, though. The grade of a cancer cell can be high or low. Low-grade cells are not likely to grow and are not a cause for concern, whereas high-grade cells are more likely to proliferate and spread.

risk elements

While the actual cause of prostate cancer is unknown, the following risk factors may increase the likelihood that it may occur:

Age: Prostate cancer is uncommon before the age of 45, although the risk increases after 50.

Black people experience the condition more frequently than white people do. The risk is lower for Asian and Hispanic persons than for Black or White people.

Family history: A person's risk of having prostate cancer is increased if they have close relatives who have had the disease in the past.

genetic influences The risk may be increased by inherited traits, such as modifications to the BRCA1 and BRCA2 genes. Breast cancer risk is also increased by certain gene mutations. The risk of prostate and other cancers is increased in men who were born with Lynch syndrome.

Diet: Some proof

According to a reliable source, eating a lot of fat may make you more likely to develop prostate cancer.

Added potential factors

Other variables that may affect the risk of prostate cancer include the following, though further research is required to validate their influence:

obesity, smoking, drinking, being exposed to chemicals like the herbicide Agent Orange, prostate inflammation, and sexually transmitted diseases

vasectomy procedure

Facts About Prostate Infections You Should Know

Only a small portion of men with prostatitis have prostate infections. Acute and chronic prostatic infections make up this minor portion.

Most acute and chronic prostatic infections are brought on by E. coli and other Gram-negative bacteria.

Groin pain, dysuria, pain during ejaculation, and decreased urine production are all signs of prostate infection. Other symptoms may include fever, lethargy, and repeated recurrence of symptoms even after therapy.

If symptoms appear, seek medical attention. If fever or inability to urinate occurs, seek emergency care.

Identification of the agent (the great majority of which are bacteria) infecting the prostate allows for the diagnosis of prostate infections or prostatitis.

Antibiotics are typically used to treat prostate infections or prostatitis; severe infections may necessitate hospitalization and intravenous antibiotic therapy for chronic infectious prostatitis.

Home care is only for pain management. Men who have prostatitis or a prostate infection require medical attention.

It's crucial to follow up to make sure the therapy was effective or to plan additional care in case the illness reappears.

Some prostate infections cannot be avoided, however, you can lessen your chances of developing infectious prostatitis by avoiding groin trauma or injury, sexually transmitted diseases, and dehydration.

Acute infectious prostatitis typically has an excellent prognosis, but chronic infectious prostatitis has a fair prognosis due to its challenging treatment.

Why do Prostate Infections Occur

Only a small portion of prostatitis instances are brought on by bacterial infections. The reason for the remaining percent of cases, which are either caused by the chronic pelvic pain syndrome or the asymptomatic inflammatory prostatitis mentioned above, is unknown. For both acute and chronic infectious prostatitis, the following prostate infectious agents are present:

The germ that causes prostate infections most frequently is Escherichia coli (E Coli), and about 80% of bacterial pathogens are gram-negative organisms (for example, Escherichia coli, Enterobacter, Serratia, Pseudomonas, Enterococcus, and Proteus species).

The most frequently identified species are Chlamydia, Neisseria, Trichomonas, and Ureaplasma. Sexually transmitted disease-causing organisms can also cause infectious prostatitis, especially in sexually active men under the age of 35.

Infrequently, diverse species like fungus, genital viruses, and parasites have been implicated, as have staphylococcal and streptococcal organisms.

There are two basic ways that the infectious agent (often bacteria) might enter the prostate.

Through the prostatic ducts, germs from a prior urethral infection enter the prostate (occasionally termed retrograde infection).

Through the ejaculatory channels, contaminated urine can spread to the glandular prostate tissue and cause infection (occasionally termed antegrade infection).

As previously mentioned, two of the four basic kinds of prostatitis—chronic infectious prostatitis and acute infectious prostatitis—are caused by infectious organisms.

Typical prostate issues include

benign prostatic hyperplasia (BPH), an enlarged prostate caused by something other than cancer, prostatitis, inflammation or swelling of the prostate, and prostate cancer

What causes issues with the prostate?

The potential root cause of prostate issues is

prostatitis\sBPH

Your doctor might not always be able to pinpoint the precise source of your prostate issue.

Prostatitis

Whether you have bacterial or chronic prostatitis will determine the etiology of your condition.

persistent prostatitis Chronic prostatitis' precise cause is unknown to medical professionals. According to researchers, persistent prostatitis might be brought on by an infection with microscopic organisms rather than bacteria. Other possible causes include chemicals in your urine, a past UTI's bodily reaction, or nerve damage in your pelvic region. In most cases, men with chronic prostatitis have no infection, according to experts.

bacteria-related prostatitis Some types of prostatitis are caused by bacteria, which are microscopic organisms that can cause an infection.

Prostatic Hyperplasia in Men

Doctors are unsure of BPH's actual cause. BPH may be brought on by alterations in the levels of the male hormone in older men, aging, inflammation, and fibrosis. When excess tissue accumulates and thickens and stiffens around your organs, it's called fibrosis.

Who gets prostate issues and how frequently do they occur

Any male can experience prostate issues. Men of all ages can develop prostate cancer. However, in men under 50, it is the most typical prostate issue. The most frequent prostate issue in males over 50 is BPH.

Prostatitis

You can be more susceptible to developing bacterial prostatitis if you have a UTI. You may be more susceptible to developing chronic prostatitis if you have lower urinary tract nerve damage or are under mental stress.

Prostatic Hyperplasia in Men

Rarely do men under the age of 40 exhibit BPH symptoms. Men who have BPH symptoms are more prevalent as they age.

BPH may be more likely to affect you if it runs in your family. Certain medical disorders and way of life decisions may also increase your risk for BPH.

hepatic hemangioma

Atangled web of blood vessels within or on the surface of the liver is known as liver hemangioma. Noncancerous and typically causing no symptoms, this tumor. Most people don't even realize they have liver hemangiomas, in fact. The majority of the time, it is only identified through a test or operation for another condition. The majority of hepatic hemangiomas don't need treatment, even after being identified.

Since liver hemangiomas are benign, they don't raise your risk of getting cancer. The tumor is typically tiny, with a diameter of fewer than 4 millimeters. But occasionally, it might expand significantly. Abdominal pain and nausea are among the symptoms that a bigger tumor is more likely to produce. Large hemangiomas are more likely to occur in pregnant women and women taking estrogen replacement therapy. This is due to the possibility that estrogen may aid in the development of hepatic **hemangiomas**. Most patients only have one hemangioma in their liver. The liver, however, can develop many hemangiomas at once.

In adults, hepatic hemangiomas normally don't result in difficulties, but when they appear in infants, they can be more harmful. The growth in infants is known as infantile **hemangioendothelioma**. Typically, it is discovered before the infant turns 6 months old. In babies, this is a rare condition. Despite not being malignant, the growth has been associated with an increased risk of heart failure.

survival for stage 4 colon cancer

Colon cancer that has metastasized to other tissues and organs is considered to be in stage 4 of the disease. The liver is where colon cancer most frequently metastasizes, however it can also move to the lungs, lymph nodes, or the lining of the abdominal cavity.

The 5-year relative survival rate for persons with stage 4 colon cancer that has spread is 14%, according to the American Cancer Society (ACS)Trusted Source.

Everyone is unique, though, and other elements affect a person's chance of surviving.

What is colon cancer in stage 4?

As the name suggests, colon cancer is any cancer affecting the colon, the last segment of the human gastrointestinal system that includes the rectum and anus. It is commonly classed alongside other cancers of the large intestine as "colorectal cancer." Colon cancer, like other cancers, isn't just one disease; it's a collection of diseases of a specific sort that affect a particular place (you can compare this to the common cold, an upper respiratory tract infection). The upper respiratory tract is affected by a number of different viral and occasionally bacterial illnesses that collectively make up the common cold. Adenocarcinoma, or cancer of the mucous-producing glands, is the most typical type of colon cancer. You may also be familiar with this term as the most typical type of lung and pancreatic cancer. Squamous cell carcinomas, GI stromal tumors, and soft-tissue sarcomas that affect the connective tissues holding your intestines in place are less prevalent forms of colon cancer.

Colon cancer is staged based on the size, penetration, and, most importantly, the spread of cancer (the Canadian Cancer

Society has a great resource for a full explanation of colon cancer staging). The Canadian Cancer Society has information on the stages of colorectal cancer (https://www.cancer.ca/en/cancer-information/cancer-type/colorectal/staging/?region=on). Any cancer that has "distant metastasis," or spread to distant organs and tissues, is said to be in stage IV. Why is...

Do stage 3 colon cancer patients have a high likelihood of passing away?

No. I still exist ten years after being diagnosed with Stage 3 colon cancer. An outstanding colorectal surgeon did my procedure. I believe that—not a general surgeon, but a colorectal surgeon—was the secret to my survival. The standard colon cancer chemotherapy followed. Still around and doing well.

Many adults in their 70s and 80s receive a colon cancer diagnosis.

What is the ideal course of action for colon cancer in stage 4

Generally speaking, one should confirm the diagnosis. A biopsy of a metastatic focus may be necessary depending on the situation because not all scan abnormalities are malignancies.

The majority of stage 4 colon cancers can be treated to lessen symptoms and extend life. Multi-drug chemotherapy regimens including FOLFIRI, FOLFOX, and XELOX are among the common chemotherapy treatments. These can occasionally be used with the angiogenesis inhibitor Avastin (bevacizumab). The majority of the time, the treatments are well tolerated. If EGFR-targeting antibodies can be employed in the future can be determined by KRAS mutation testing.

With targeted therapy to a relatively small number of liver or lung metastases, some stage 4 colon cancers may be curable. This may involve doing surgery to remove the metastasis, or it may involve combining the aforementioned treatments with radiofrequency ablation, cryotherapy, or stereotactic radiosurgery.

renal cancer

One type of cancer that develops in the kidneys is known as kidney cancer. The abdomen houses a pair of organs called the kidneys. Urine is created after they filter blood waste. Both the right and left kidneys are susceptible to developing kidney cancer.

Renal cell carcinoma (RCC) and transitional cell carcinoma are the two main kinds of kidney cancer (TCC). Approximately 80% of kidney malignancies are RCCs. TCC is less frequent, making up only 15% of cases. The remaining cases of kidney cancer are rare subtypes called sarcomas and lymphomas.

Most persons with kidney cancer in its early stages don't have any symptoms. Typically, the cancer is discovered by chance during a CT scan or MRI that was done for another purpose. Cancer symptoms, such as hematuria (blood in the urine), back or side discomfort, exhaustion, and weight loss, may worsen as the disease progresses. Please visit your doctor straight away if you have any of these symptoms. Typically, it is an advanced stage of cancer when symptoms appear.

renal cancer warning signs

Blood in the pee; a tumor or lump near your kidneys.
    -A general feeling of being unwell.
    -Appetite loss.
    -Losing weight.
    -Bone ache.
    -A lot of calcium.
    -Fatigue.
    - Unaccounted-for weight loss
    -A persistent fever that is not brought on by an infection.

Hepatomegaly

Hepatomegaly is an overly inflated liver, which means it is larger than typical.

Your liver performs numerous crucial tasks. By getting rid of toxic compounds that your body produces, it helps to purify your blood. It produces bile, a fluid that aids in digesting dietary fat. Additionally, it stores glucose, a type of sugar that provides an instant energy boost when required.

Typically, an enlarged liver is a sign of another illness, such as hepatitis. There are several available treatments, but you must first identify the underlying source of the issue.

Symptoms of Hepatomegaly

Usually, if your liver is somewhat enlarged, you won't have any symptoms. Depending on how large it is, you might have:
- A sensation of satiety
- Burning in your stomach

You can have symptoms depending on the cause of your enlarged liver.

-Tannification of the skin or eyes (jaundice)
   -Weakness and fatigue
   -Nausea -Loss of weight

What causes hepatomegaly?

Hepatomegaly can be caused by a variety of factors.

infections, fatty deposits, storage issues, and hepatic vascular problems
   Tumors and bowel obstruction
   -Liver cysts - Genetic and autoimmune disorders.